Generis
PUBLISHING

Building Tomorrow's Healthcare in the DRC

Blueprint for a Modern, Humane, and Functional Medical System in the Heart of Africa

Samuel Mulumba Ntafua

Title: Building Tomorrow's Healthcare in the DRC

Blueprint for a Modern, Humane, and Functional Medical System in the Heart of Africa

ISBN: 979-8-89966-651-3

Author: Samuel Mulumba Ntafua

Cover image: https://pixabay.com/

Publisher: Generis Publishing
Online orders: www.generis-publishing.com
Contact email: info@generis-publishing.com

DEDICATION

To the memory of my father, Nkongolo Muila Tshibola, whose silent wisdom remains by my side, like a modest but ever-present star.

To my mother, Véronique Tshibola, for her unconditional love, her constancy in prayer, and her unfailing presence during the crucial moments of my life.

To Papa François Mupepe and Maman Silvie Kayowa, I wish to express my gratitude for your warm welcome, your affectionate support, and the precious blessings you offered me during the decisive steps of my journey.

To my wife, Patricia Mupepe Ntafua, whose profound serenity and essential presence bring me the balance I need so much every day. Your soothing calm, your constant light, your discreet but essential presence... you are the silent root of my harmony.

To Hadriel and Crystal-Amalia, this book is dedicated to you as a symbol of hope. May you discover in it the strength and inspiration necessary to build a fairer and more humane future.

May these pages bear witness to authentic love, lasting commitment, and a call for collective responsibility.

ACKNOWLEDGMENTS

First and foremost, I pay tribute to God, the source of life and inspiration, to whom the origin as well as the completion of this project belongs.

I wish to express my sincere gratitude to Professor Frederic Bontango Kweme, companion of reflections and convictions, whose wise perspective, unwavering patience, and discreet support enriched my thinking far beyond this manuscript.

To my brothers and sisters, whose silent love and unceasing prayers constituted a precious support. To Jean Paul Mukolo Nkokesha, for the relevance of his words, always spoken at the right moment.

I also wish to thank the André Kadima Foundation and the late Papa André, with whom I shared dreams of a more equitable health system for the DRC, the echo of which still resonates in these pages.

Finally, to all those who have supported this project since its inception: you have not only accompanied a book, you have carried a vision.

PREFACE

This book goes beyond the framework of a simple technical essay; it serves simultaneously as an alert, a profound reflection on the healthcare challenges of the Congo, and an invitation to envision a future imbued with dignity.

In the Democratic Republic of the Congo, the healthcare issue goes far beyond logistics. It highlights our deep social inequalities, while nurturing the hope for a new social contract based on human dignity.

This text does not limit itself to establishing a clinical observation: it offers a clear path, developed from concrete realities such as overcrowded hospitals, neglected rural areas, and families in search of care. It is addressed not only to decision-makers and health professionals, but also to every citizen, because public health cannot be the exclusive preserve of experts.

Every successful reform constitutes an act of justice. Every abandonment represents a human tragedy. It is time to gather our strengths to build a health system that heals, unites, and honors.

Professor Frederic Bontango Kweme

PhD in Public Health, Leadership & Management

AUTHOR'S NOTE

I have practiced medicine under extreme clinical conditions: where care is delivered by flashlight, where diagnoses are made without any baseline diagnostics, and where a simple supply chain failure can determine life or death.

I have witnessed colleagues performing clinical miracles in degrading contexts, while patients succumbed, not to their pathologies, but due to a total lack of essential resources.

However, I have also discovered another aspect of my country: that of a resilient, inventive people who continue to fight relentlessly against adversity. It is within this permanent tension between suffering and hope that this work was born.

I did not write this as a mere observer, but as an engaged actor, firmly convinced that we can and must do better. We must redesign our healthcare delivery, optimize our resource allocation, and watch over one another.

This book is a call for rigorous, patient clinical work, anchored in our local realities. It does not offer imported solutions, but pleads for the necessity of constructing a Congolese healthcare model, designed and executed by the Congolese people themselves.

Samuel Mulumba Ntafua, MD, MPH
Public Health Specialist Physician

SYNOPSIS

Shaping Tomorrow's Healthcare in the DRC

A Practical, People-Centered Blueprint for Transformation

The Democratic Republic of the Congo stands at a critical crossroads. In the face of rapid population growth, pronounced social inequalities, and a fragile healthcare infrastructure, a comprehensive system overhaul is essential. Nevertheless, amid this complexity, a certainty persists: transformation is not only achievable, but it is also deeply urgent.

This book does not intend to be just another administrative report. It represents an act of faith in the capacity of the Congolese people to design an equitable, resilient healthcare system tailored to their specific epidemiological and social needs. Built from concrete field experience, driven by baseline values such as dignity, equity, and justice, and founded on practical proposals, this text constitutes a genuine call to action.

It speaks to decision-makers ready to initiate bold structural changes, to healthcare providers in search of professional purpose, and to all citizens convinced that health should never be a privilege reserved for the few. This text aims to be both a compass and a starting point. It calls us to build, starting today, a health system worthy of our national aspirations.

TABLE OF CONTENTS

GENERAL INTRODUCTION **13**
PART I: DIAGNOSTIC OF SYSTEMIC DYSFUNCTIONS **15**
An Analysis Structured Around Five Critical Dimensions 15
Chapter 1: Rapid Population Growth vs. Overburdened Infrastructure **17**
Demographic Pressure on a System in Crisis 17
Healthcare Planning Bereft of Concrete Data 17
Manifest Regional and Structural Imbalances 17
A Multifaceted Operational Crisis 18
An Absence of Zoning Approaching Injustice 18
Changing Direction: Thinking Locally, Acting Strategically 19
Activating Immediate Operational Levers 19
Chapter 2: Degraded Infrastructure and Missing Clinical Equipment **20**
Delivering Care without Tools: The Invisible Reality of Health Professionals ... 20
Buildings Unfit for Public Health Missions 20
The Scarcity and Non-Existence of Medical Devices 20
The Total Absence of Biomedical Engineering and Maintenance 21
Reforming the Care Environment: An Essential Priority 21
Ensuring Sustainability: Building a Resilient Network 22
Chapter 3: Disparities in Clinical Quality and Absence of Standards **23**
When Mere Access to a Facility Does Not Guarantee Care 23
Multi-Tier Medicine: The Reflection of a Fragmented System 23
Reaffirming and Systematizing Clinical Quality 24
Structuring Quality Assurance through Systemic Mechanisms 25
Chapter 4: The Healthcare Workforce Crisis: A Pillar in Distress **26**
When Medicine is Sustained by Sheer Human Endurance 26
A Professional Life under Permanent Financial and Emotional Stress 26
Valuing Clinicians: Placing Human Capital at the Center of Strategy 27
Concrete Operational Levers to Resolve the Workforce Crisis 27
Chapter 5: Insufficient and Inequitable Healthcare Financing Models **29**
When Disease Conveys Immediate Economic Ruin 29
An Unstable, Fragmented, and Profoundly Inequitable Model 29
Concrete Financial Instruments to Deploy Solidarity 31
PART II: A VISION FOR A MODERN HEALTH SYSTEM **33**
The Foundations of an Endogenous and Pragmatic Blueprint 33
A Coherent Architecture for Lasting Systemic Change 34
Chapter 6: Establishing Nationwide Territorial Equity and Access **36**
Territorial Justice: The Absolute Foundation of a Democratic Health System 36

A Fragmented Health System Operating at Multiple Speeds 36
Constructing a Health Network Rooted in Spatial Equity 37
Solid Operational Tools for Sustainable Territorial Realignment......................... 38
Chapter 7: Reinventing Medicine: Quality, Technology, and Protocol Standardization.. 40
A Technological Paradox Exposing an Institutional Emergency......................... 40
Severe Technical Deficits Conveying Heavy Human Costs 40
Deploying Frugal, Human-Centered Medical Technology.................................. 41
An Adaptable National Technological and Engineering Blueprint...................... 42
Chapter 8: Empowering Human Resources: Training, Status, and Recognition.. 44
The Human Capital: The Forgotten Foundation of Healthcare Delivery 44
Structural Vulnerabilities in Human Resource Management............................... 44
A Comprehensive Revaluation of the Healthcare Workforce.............................. 45
Solid Institutional Frameworks for Lasting Career Transformation 46
Chapter 9: Universal Health Coverage and Financial Solidarity 48
Escaping the Deep Injustice of Direct Out-of-Pocket Payments 48
When Access to Healthcare Operates as a Blind Social Lottery.......................... 48
Rebuilding Healthcare around the Core Engine of Solidarity............................. 49
The Architecture of the Universal Health Insurance System (ASURDC)............ 49
A Progressive, Transparent, and Participatory Deployment Plan........................ 50
A Project of National Society, Not a Mere Bureaucratic Adjustment.................. 51
PART III: STRUCTURAL IMPLEMENTATION BLUEPRINT 53
The Four Absolute Non-Negotiable Conditions for Lasting Reform................... 53
Activating the Four Primary Operational Levers for Execution 54
Chapter 10: Governance, Applied Research, and Change Leadership 55
Building an Accountable and Transformative Governance Framework 55
Strategic Change Leadership as the Engine of Operational Efficiency................ 55
Deep Structural Faults within the Current Governance Apparatus 56
Reconstructing Strategic Governance to Meet Continental Challenges............... 56
A Robust Scientific and Data Infrastructure as a Catalyst for Change................. 57
Repositioning the Citizen at the Absolute Center of Health Governance 58
GENERAL CONCLUSION: REDESIGNING HEALTH, REBUILDING THE NATION 59
BIBLIOGRAPHICAL REFERENCES... 63

GENERAL INTRODUCTION

The Democratic Republic of the Congo is often perceived as a waking giant. Its vast natural resources, rich landscapes, and the vitality of its youth bear witness to immense potential. Yet, behind this promising facade hides a darker, less visible, but deeply concerning reality: our healthcare system is in critical condition. From isolated rural sectors to overcrowded metropolitan hubs, millions of families live in permanent anxiety. Daily, they face heart-wrenching trade-offs: whether to purchase life-saving medicine or feed their children. This dilemma, far from being anecdotal, dictates the survival of millions of Congolese citizens.

In certain health facilities, women give birth illuminated only by a mobile phone screen. In others, nurses continue to deliver clinical care without receiving salaries, without essential medical supplies, and sometimes without any formal state recognition. As a frontline physician, I have been a direct witness to this suffering. I have delivered medical care in unacceptable environments, illuminated solely by a pocket flashlight. I have seen pregnant women lose their lives, not due to the clinical complexity of their condition, but simply because there was no available cesarean kit, no blood unit for transfusion, or no operational medical transport to evacuate them in time.

These deaths, though entirely preventable, cannot be attributed to fate. They raise a fundamental institutional question: why do the leaders of our country choose to seek medical treatment abroad? Above all, what message does this medical flight send to those who have no choice but to survive within a broken system?

The current crisis is not merely epidemiological or clinical. It is profoundly moral, because it exposes our collective failure to protect the most vulnerable. It is social, revealing flagrant inequities. And it is deeply political, underscoring the absence of long-term strategic vision in public health management.

However, despite this alarming picture, reasons for hope endure. Our frontline healthcare workers demonstrate exceptional courage. Local communities organize, innovate, and resist. The youth, driven by a desire for sustainable change, constitute a powerful force. What is still lacking is a clear direction, an assertive political will, and a coherent strategy capable of building a truly functional health system.

It is this urgency that inspired this book. It rests on a profound conviction: health must not be a privilege reserved for an elite. It represents a fundamental human right, a core requirement of dignity, and an unavoidable lever for national development. It is time to end stopgap measures and transcend superficial reforms. What the Democratic Republic of the Congo requires today is a deep structural transformation—thoughtful, organized, and resolutely ambitious.

Our methodology is structured around a simple yet rigorous analytical framework: Problem-Result-System (PRS). Each chapter identifies a concrete dysfunction observed on the ground, defines the target clinical or social results to be achieved, and then proposes realistic, localized action mechanisms. There is no technocratic jargon or illusory promises, but rather a functional roadmap anchored in Congolese reality. This project addresses those who, at various levels of leadership, wish to act without further delay. It challenges healthcare professionals who refuse to yield to resignation. Finally, it addresses all those who still believe in the power of collective commitment to rebuild a nation. The DRC possesses the human, social, and cultural capital necessary to become a public health model on the African continent. The time to act is not in the future; it is already here. This transformation begins now, through a lucid acknowledgment of our failures, a shared vision for the future, and a shared determination to rebuild a health system worthy of its name.

PART I:

DIAGNOSTIC OF SYSTEMIC DYSFUNCTIONS

Analyzing Vulnerabilities to Build Better Healthcare Delivery

Any meaningful reform of a healthcare system begins with a crucial and non-negotiable step: clearly recognizing its deepest structural weaknesses. Before designing reconstruction strategies, it is imperative to identify exactly what requires correction, interrogate the existing operational foundations, and respond appropriately to the clinical realities observed on the ground.

This first section presents a rigorous analysis of the current state of the health system in the Democratic Republic of the Congo. It is intended neither as an indictment nor as a simple collection of grievances, but rather as an investigation anchored in the lived experiences of patients, frontline clinicians, healthcare administrators, and community leaders. Through their challenges, but also their ingenuity and resilience, a precise mapping of current operational dysfunctions emerges.

Indeed, healing a sick system requires more than statistical aggregates or abstract technical theories. It implies understanding how, on a daily basis, chronic supply shortages, arbitrary administrative decisions, and hesitant governance directly impact the real health outcomes of the Congolese people. This diagnostic framework targets four principal objectives: it aims to offer a realistic and contextualized reading of the current health system, removed from theoretical approaches disconnected from local realities; it highlights the structural barriers hindering healthcare access, compromising safety, and limiting equity and clinical efficacy; it illustrates the interlacing factors between rapid demographic growth, weak training systems, opaque governance, and inequitable financing; and finally, it aspires to trigger a collective awareness capable of breaking the spiral of resignation and opening the way for meaningful legislative and structural reforms.

An Analysis Structured Around Five Critical Dimensions

The chosen approach rests on an in-depth thematic analysis, broken down into five chapters, each focused on a fundamental driver of the current crisis:

• **Chapter 1** examines the impact of rapid population growth and the organizational disorder of health services. In two decades, the Congolese population has doubled without a parallel evolution in healthcare capacity, leaving cities saturated and rural areas neglected due to a lack of territorial planning.

• **Chapter 2** focuses on the critical state of medical infrastructure and the alarming scarcity of available diagnostics and clinical tools, turning medical delivery into an act of basic survival for both staff and patients.

• **Chapter 3** addresses the issue of healthcare quality, which is often left to individual discretion in the absence of clear clinical guidelines, protocols, or reliable quality assurance mechanisms, compromising patient safety.

• **Chapter 4** highlights the healthcare workforce crisis, characterized by widespread clinician burnout, erratic salary payouts, and precarious working conditions.

• **Chapter 5** deals with financing models. In a country where poverty remains endemic, the financial burden rests almost exclusively on households in the absence of institutional risk-pooling or solidarity mechanisms.

Together, these elements reveal a system under permanent distress: underfunded, fragmented, poorly regulated, and structurally incapable of meeting population demands. These are not isolated issues; they interlock and reinforce each other, rendering partial or strictly technical answers ineffective. What the DRC needs is a genuine paradigm shift that anchors all transformation in our local socio-epidemiological realities for the general public interest.

Chapter 1:

Rapid Population Growth vs. Overburdened Infrastructure

Demographic Pressure on a System in Crisis

Currently, the Democratic Republic of the Congo faces one of the fastest demographic expansion rates globally. With a population approaching one hundred million inhabitants, the majority of whom are under the age of 25, the country possesses a considerable human asset. Nevertheless, this youth population, which could serve as a vector for national transformation, collides directly with the persistent fragility of health infrastructures. This growing imbalance between rapidly increasing healthcare demands and the system's capacity to respond exerts significant stress across the entire national medical network.

Over the last twenty years, the population has doubled, whereas the number of operational clinical facilities, qualified professionals, and material resources has not experienced any proportional increase. This manifest mismatch illustrates a historical inability to anticipate social evolutions, further weakening an already struggling healthcare apparatus.

Healthcare Planning Bereft of Concrete Data

Effective healthcare planning relies fundamentally on reliable demographic and epidemiological data: it is crucial to know our population size, geographic distribution, and specific clinical needs based on regional variations. Yet, this essential information is largely missing from central decision-making processes. Healthcare capacity remains stagnant while the population grows, budgets do not progress realistically, staff allocations are frequently arbitrary, and infrastructural investments continue to concentrate heavily in major cities to the complete detriment of rural health zones.

Manifest Regional and Structural Imbalances

On the ground, signs of organizational failure are omnipresent. In Kisangani, a single midwife may find herself supervising multiple complex deliveries simultaneously. In Sankuru, children must walk more than twenty kilometers to obtain a simple medical consultation. In Kinshasa, tertiary referral hospitals are so overwhelmed that patient queues extend into the streets.

Although a pyramidal healthcare referral model is theoretically established, it is functionally inverted. Primary care health centers, intended to be the first point of care for patients, are routinely neglected, under- equipped, or completely non-operational. Consequently, patients bypass them, forcing saturated secondary and tertiary reference hospitals to manage primary care burdens they are neither staffed nor funded to support. This generates a structural collapse: peripheral facilities empty out while urban medical centers are heavily congested.

A Multifaceted Operational Crisis

Each year, more than three million births are recorded across the nation. However, rural maternity wards lack basic beds, qualified personnel, and essential neonatal equipment. This overcrowding leads to preventable obstetric complications and maternal mortality, alongside a progressive deterioration of working conditions and profound professional burnout among clinicians.

Territorial inequalities are widening. Certain provinces, such as Kasaï or Maniema, contain entire localities that have not seen a physician in years. Meanwhile, Kinshasa alone concentrates over 60% of the country's healthcare professionals, deepening regional disparities. Furthermore, the youth demographic generates specific health needs that remain largely ignored. Critical issues relating to mental health, sexual and reproductive education, and the prevention of high-risk behaviors are rarely addressed due to a lack of trained providers and adapted clinical frameworks. A healthcare worker in Haut-Uele summarizes: "The youth want to understand, they want to ask questions, but we have neither the clinical tools nor the dedicated spaces to answer them."

An Absence of Zoning Approaching Injustice

The Congolese health system functions at multiple speeds. While major urban centers continue to attract the majority of human and financial resources, rural zones struggle to retain clinicians, stabilize basic services, and meet growing demands. This imbalance, far from being strictly technical or administrative, results from long- term political choices. When health strategy is not aligned with territorial realities, healthcare access ceases to be a constitutional right and becomes a geographical lottery. It is no longer clinical need that determines care, but one's location on a map.

Changing Direction: Thinking Locally, Acting Strategically

To remedy these structural imbalances, it is imperative to adopt proactive, flexible health planning attentive to real demographic dynamics. This requires not only tracking population movements but also forecasting future epidemiological needs and redeploying resources where they are most urgently required. It is not merely a question of mass infrastructure construction, but of designing adaptable facilities equitably distributed and capable of responding to local specificities. This should include, for example, youth-adapted health centers, mobile clinics in isolated territories, or intermediate secondary triage hubs on the peripheries of large agglomerations to alleviate pressure on central university hospitals.

Moreover, solidarity between provinces must become a tangible reality. Encouraging the retention of healthcare professionals in difficult, remote health zones requires substantial institutional incentives: attractive hardship premiums, functional staff housing, and clear opportunities for career advancement.

Activating Immediate Operational Levers

Several measures can be executed without delay to rebalance the system:

- **Dynamic Health Mapping:** Develop a digitized national health map, updated via mobile tools, to direct public and private investments based on real-time population changes and infrastructural deficits.

- **Health Equalization Fund:** Establish a healthcare financial equalization fund designed to reinforce under- resourced provinces, using objective criteria such as population density, local poverty indexes, and geographic accessibility following chapter.

Chapter 2:

Degraded Infrastructure and Missing Clinical Equipment

Delivering Care without Tools: The Invisible Reality of Health Professionals

A healthcare system cannot be reduced solely to the clinical expertise of its practitioners or the theoretical design of its public policies. It requires robust physical infrastructure, structurally safe medical installations, and adequate clinical technology. In the Democratic Republic of the Congo, these essential elements are routinely absent. In numerous health centers, medical procedures are performed by candlelight, without access to running water, and lacking the most basic medical consumables. This reality is not an exception, but rather the standard baseline across vast rural sectors of our country. This situation, often masked in generalized statistics, heavily compromises clinical safety and challenges the core bioethics of medical interventions.

Buildings Unfit for Public Health Missions

In multiple provinces, health infrastructure is in a state of physical collapse. Certain facilities are still housed in buildings dating back to the colonial era that have never undergone structural renovations. Others operate out of rented residential houses entirely unsuited for infection control or clinical workflows. The problems are pervasive: collapsing roofs, cracked walls, and patient rooms completely devoid of natural ventilation or appropriate lighting. It is common for delivery rooms to lack proper obstetric beds or for operating theatres to be completely deprived of emergency backup power. In this context, the total absence of potable water, functional sanitation, or reliable waste management systems compromises patient safety and strips away human dignity.

The Scarcity and Non-Existence of Medical Devices

Where physical structures struggle to remain standing, basic medical equipment is scarcer still. In some health centers, a single stethoscope must be shared among multiple clinicians. In others, clinical diagnoses are made entirely via visual inspection due to a total lack of basic laboratory or diagnostic reagents. Laboratories, where they exist, are severely under-equipped. Basic diagnostic imaging and resuscitation devices are critically missing, making the management of medical emergencies virtually impossible. In rural zones, a critical emergency frequently transforms into an unwritten death sentence simply because the required tools are absent. Even when emergency transport vehicles are allocated, they are routinely broken down, devoid of fuel, or diverted from their medical missions. The ambulance, which should be a tool for rapid life-saving intervention, becomes a symbol of systemic failure.

The Total Absence of Biomedical Engineering and Maintenance

Even when a hospital receives new medical devices through international donations or state procurement, these devices regularly break down without any repair mechanisms in place. The absence of a preventative maintenance plan, dedicated engineering budgets, or localized biomedical technicians creates an alarming graveyard of technology: high-tech equipment is abandoned for months or years due to minor, fixable faults. Investment without operational follow-up transforms into immediate capital loss.

Reforming the Care Environment: An Essential Priority

The response to this material crisis can no longer be delayed. It is imperative to develop infrastructure specifically adapted to our environment. These structures do not need to be complex or overly expensive, but they must be functional, easy to clean, well-ventilated, and possess reliable access to water and electricity. The integration of renewable energy, particularly solar power grids, represents the only sustainable solution for health zones disconnected from national electricity networks.

Before any acquisition of medical devices, a rigorous baseline evaluation must be conducted: Is this equipment adapted to the local climate and dust conditions? Can it be easily maintained? Is there an active local maintenance contract? It is clinically and economically illogical to procure a CT scanner if no local competency is available to repair it or operate it safely. Furthermore, an integrated emergency evacuation network must be established. Each health district should possess at least one terrain-appropriate medical transport vehicle: fully equipped 4x4 vehicles, river ambulances, or medical motorbikes. These assets must be backed by continuous community training in first aid and connected to functional local dispatch centers using a unique, free emergency number.

Finally, medical equipment asset management must be entirely digitized. Every device must be barcoded, geolocated, and tracked throughout its lifecycle. Such traceability would allow administrators to know, in real time, what is operational, what is broken down, and what requires technical intervention or immediate replacement.

Ensuring Sustainability: Building a Resilient Network

The long-term survival of health infrastructure requires solid institutional mechanisms. It is crucial to establish national architectural and engineering building codes for health facilities that take into account geographic and climatic variations, while imposing minimum quality standards on all actors, including international NGOs. A National Medical Equipment Plan (NMEP) would allow the state to census needs province by province, identify a standardized list of adapted devices for each level of care, and coordinate procurement to maximize financial mutualization and efficiency.

The development of a certified national cadre of biomedical technicians is equally indispensable. These professionals must be distributed across every province to guarantee rapid proximity maintenance, reducing dependency on the capital. Maintenance contracts must become a legally mandatory component of any medical device acquisition, featuring clear clauses regarding technical inspection frequency and localized response times. Finally, implementing an interoperable, transparent Integrated Medical Equipment Management System (IMEMS) would provide all stakeholders—the state, donors, and local health administrators—with a clear vision of park status, technical emergencies, and budgetary priorities.

We too often forget that quality of care begins with the physical space where it is delivered. A surgeon without a scalpel, a maternity ward without clean water, a hospital without power: each of these deficits transforms medicine into an impossible mission. Investing in infrastructure is not a secondary luxury; it is a matter of absolute justice, an act of respect toward clinicians, and a recognition of the fundamental rights of patients. However, improving material conditions is only half the battle. The next challenge is more subtle but equally vital: it concerns the clinical quality of practices, medical standard operating procedures, and patient safety, which will be explored in the next chapter.

Chapter 3:

Disparities in Clinical Quality and Absence of Standards

When Mere Access to a Facility Does Not Guarantee Care

In the Democratic Republic of the Congo, physically reaching a health center guarantees neither a reliable diagnosis nor an evidence-based treatment regimen. The clinical pathway of a patient presenting with the exact same pathology can vary drastically depending on whether they are treated in Mbuji-Mayi or Kinshasa. This systemic disparity is far from negligible; it highlights a deeply inequitable system where clinical quality depends on chance, location, or personal luck.

This extreme variability in patient management does not stem from the clinical severity of the pathology itself. It is dictated by factors entirely external to the patient: their place of residence, the baseline training level of the specific staff on duty, and the diagnostics available at the exact moment of consultation. This raises a crucial bioethical question that goes beyond technical metrics: how can we guarantee every Congolese citizen, regardless of socio-economic status or geography, access to safe, dignified, and evidence-based care?

Multi-Tier Medicine: The Reflection of a Fragmented System

Within our health institutions, we observe alarming variations in clinical practices, not only between different provinces but often within the walls of the exact same facility. This lack of standardization represents a severe risk to patient safety. In many cases, medical care is delivered without any adherence to national protocols. Clinical decisions rely heavily on individual provider experience, empirical habits, or immediate resource availability, rather than on robust scientific evidence and uniform guidelines.

Due to the total absence of updated clinical textbooks or accessible diagnostic algorithms, common endemic diseases—such as malaria or respiratory infections—are frequently managed via empirical knowledge transmitted orally. This operational unpredictability becomes the baseline norm in contexts where diagnostics are broken, physicians are absent, and essential drugs are out of stock. In this climate of absolute uncertainty, nurses find themselves performing complex surgical or medical acts strictly reserved for specialized physicians.

Complex deliveries are managed by unqualified auxiliary personnel, exposing mothers to fatal obstetric complications. Conversely, while a wealthy minority delivers under continuous electronic fetal monitoring in private urban clinics, rural mothers give birth by candlelight without sterile gloves or basic antiseptics. This double standard feeds a growing public mistrust in the formal health sector, driving populations toward self-medication, unqualified traditional practitioners, and complete medical abandonment.

Reaffirming and Systematizing Clinical Quality

Ensuring quality of care does not mean creating an inflexible, blind bureaucracy. It means establishing a clear, flexible, and pragmatic framework capable of safely guiding health professionals working in highly constrained environments. Simple protocols, written in accessible language, tailored to local epidemiological realities and regularly updated, must form the foundation of this normalization.

These clinical guidelines must be disseminated across multiple formats: printed booklets, wallcharts posted in clinical spaces, offline-accessible mobile applications, and routine SMS alerts, ensuring they reach providers working in zones entirely cut off from the internet. The objective is to provide clinicians with practical, actionable tools: standardized partographs for delivery monitoring, clear diagnostic algorithms, and baseline infection control checklists. This operational framework safeguards clinical practice while reducing the massive gap in care quality between urban and rural facilities.

To oversee this transition, creating a National Agency for Healthcare Quality Assessment (NAHQA) could serve as a powerful institutional lever. This independent entity would be tasked with conducting regular clinical audits, tracking key performance indicators (such as maternal mortality or post-operative infection rates), and publishing transparent public reports. Over time, state and donor funding for health structures should be explicitly linked not just to their administrative existence, but to verified clinical quality outcomes on the ground. Instilling a culture of continuous quality improvement is paramount: regular training, systematic mortality reviews (maternal and neonatal death audits) after every serious adverse event, and the progressive implementation of electronic medical records are vital mechanisms to foster collective learning and prevent the repetition of avoidable medical errors.

Structuring Quality Assurance through Systemic Mechanisms

To ensure these quality initiatives endure over time, a coherent institutional ecosystem must be built:

- **National Accreditation Framework:** Establish a transparent national accreditation system that grades health facilities based on verified safety and quality metrics, directly impacting their licensing and public funding tiers.

- **Congolese Clinical Guidelines Committee:** Form an active scientific committee to design realistic, evidence-based guidelines tailored to resource-constrained environments.

- **Continuous Quality Dashboards:** Implementation of real-time quality monitoring tools focusing on simple, high-impact metrics: nosocomial infection rates, patient triage times, and verified patient satisfaction scores.

- **Dedicated Quality Officers:** Appoint and train a dedicated healthcare quality officer within each health zone to oversee protocol adherence, manage continuous on-the-job training, and report local operational difficulties back to central levels.

Finally, baseline medical and nursing education must integrate these quality and safety standards from day one. The emergence of provincial quality mentors, peer-review networks, and shared digital libraries will facilitate the collective ownership of these practices, transforming quality assurance from a top-down bureaucratic burden into an internalized clinical reflex.

Trust is the ultimate foundation of any therapeutic relationship. It emerges from a respectful reception, attentive listening, and consistent care. These clinical interactions, though hard to quantify, are what encourage a patient to adhere to a treatment regimen, return for follow-up, or recommend a health facility to their family. However, this trust is intrinsically fragile; it degrades with every instance of negligence, every avoidable error, health reform.

Chapter 4:

The Healthcare Workforce Crisis: A Pillar in Distress

When Medicine is Sustained by Sheer Human Endurance

The physical walls of a health facility do not guarantee the healing of patients. Even with state-of-the-art infrastructure and advanced diagnostic tools, a health system remains completely inert without the human beings who animate it. Physicians, nurses, midwives, laboratory technicians, community health officers, cleaners, and administrative clerks form the backbone of our healthcare delivery. Their daily commitment is the ultimate determinant of quality. Yet, this essential human capital is currently experiencing a severe, chronic crisis. Systematically excluded from high-level policy decisions, under-resourced in their daily practice, and stripped of basic professional dignity, our healthcare workforce suffers from profound, structural exhaustion. This chapter investigates the root causes of this systemic distress, not to assign blame, but to identify realistic structural levers for transformation.

A Professional Life under Permanent Financial and Emotional Stress

Absolute precariousness has become the baseline norm for Congolese healthcare workers. Salaries, when paid at all, arrive with severe delays and remain well below a livable wage. Formal social safety nets are non- existent, and the prospect of a dignified retirement remains a distant illusion. It is common to encounter frontline physicians working for consecutive months without receiving a single paycheck, or nurses forced to work multiple jobs simultaneously across different clinics, heavily compromising their own health and clinical safety.

Faced with this absolute financial insecurity, many clinicians see no alternative but to demand direct payments from patients prior to delivering care, dangerously blurring the line between public service and basic economic survival. While this practice is an understandable survival mechanism within the current broken framework, it deeply fractures the therapeutic relationship of trust with patients and erects an insuperable financial barrier to care. To this financial precariousness is added a total lack of professional recognition. In isolated territories, a rural midwife may save multiple lives every week without ever receiving a formal administrative acknowledgment, a clear promotion pathway, or access to continuous medical education. To specialize or advance professionally, clinicians must abandon their rural communities to move to Kinshasa or go abroad—an option restricted to a wealthy minority. This toxic environment drives talent away from the public sector. Some defect to international NGOs, others move entirely into private practice, and the most disillusioned abandon the medical profession altogether.

Valuing Clinicians: Placing Human Capital at the Center of Strategy

To reconstruct our national health system, we must radically redefine the role of the healthcare worker, viewing them not as mere administrative executors but as strategic actors of national development. They are the drivers of clinical innovation, the guardians of medical ethics, and the visible link between the state and the citizen. This recognition must manifest through concrete structural measures: dignified, regular salaries, paired with clear hardship premiums for those practicing in remote or conflict-affected health zones, clear employment contracts, and comprehensive occupational health insurance. The institutional message must be simple: "Your work is essential, therefore your life and livelihood are protected."

However, professional revaluation cannot be limited to financial remuneration. It must include clear, transparent career advancement pathways. This requires decentralized continuous medical education accessible at the provincial level, allowing for specialization without forcing clinicians to resign from their rural posts.

Furthermore, staff allocations must be managed humanely. Dispatching a young medical graduate to an isolated, enclaved region without providing basic housing, access to schools for their children, or healthcare for their own family is an administrative failure that guarantees their immediate departure. Conversely, providing decent housing, family support envelopes, and transport assistance transforms an administrative obligation into a sustainable professional choice. Finally, healthcare workers must be actively included in the governance systems that dictate their practice. Involving them in local co-management, publicly celebrating clinical successes, and collectively auditing systemic failures are vital steps to restore a culture of mutual respect.

Concrete Operational Levers to Resolve the Workforce Crisis

To translate these strategic ambitions into reality, specific operational mechanisms must be deployed:

• **Unified National Salary Scale:** Implement a clear, transparent national salary grid based on objective metrics: verified qualifications, years of experience, actual job function, regional hardship tier, and documented monthly clinical hours, eliminating opaque local negotiations.

• **Rural Retention Package:** Design a comprehensive statutory retention package for remote health zones that combines substantial financial premiums, guaranteed functional housing, education stipends for children, and prioritized access to post-graduate specialization scholarships after a completed rural tenure.

• **Mobile Medical Volunteer Brigades:** Organize structured, state-supported mobile brigades of volunteer clinicians to temporarily reinforce enclaved health zones during epidemiological surges or acute staffing shortages, backed by robust logistics and strict rotational schedules.

• **National Institute for Continuous Professional Development:** Found a dedicated national institute utilizing hybrid learning methodologies (mobile offline platforms, localized peer tutoring, and practical provincial workshops) to deliver continuous education, backed by a mandatory Continuing Professional Development (CPD) credit tracking system.

• **Digital Career Management Platform:** Modernize human resource operations through a transparent, centralized digital platform co-managed with health unions and professional orders, ensuring all appointments, promotions, and transfers are fully traceable and merit-based.

We must remember that for the vast majority of Congolese citizens, the visible face of the state is neither a central minister nor a member of parliament; it is the village nurse or the district physician. If this professional is neglected, demoralized, and abandoned by institutions, the message transmitted to our population is clear: "Your life does not matter." A disconnected, disengaged healthcare worker is not a traitor to their Hippocratic oath; they are the direct reflection of a system that has betrayed them. Restoring a human, predictable, and equitable management of our health workforce is not a secondary administrative task. It is a profound ethical which will be scrutinized in the next chapter.

Chapter 5:

Insufficient and Inequitable Healthcare Financing Models

When Disease Conveys Immediate Economic Ruin

In the Democratic Republic of the Congo, accessing medical care remains inextricably tied to a painful, omnipresent question: "Do I have the money?" This inquiry, which should be entirely obsolete in an equitable society, highlights a profound structural defect: the constitutional right to health is systematically subverted by immediate financial barriers. Consequently, millions of Congolese citizens find themselves trapped in an unacceptable cycle of physical suffering, deep economic precariousness, and medical care renunciation, bearing a double burden that is both clinical and financial.

In this broken framework, even a minor medical intervention can trigger catastrophic household expenditure and deep social exclusion. Due to the chronic deficit in public healthcare subsidies, medical facilities are forced to operate as commercial entities, recovering all operational costs directly from patients. The price of a simple dressing, a routine consult, or a normal delivery transforms into an insuperable financial obstacle. This forces the most vulnerable to dangerously delay seeking care, resort to informal and dangerous parallel markets, or completely abandon any hope of treatment. The current financing model silently condemns the poorest to pay with their health, and frequently, with their lives.

An Unstable, Fragmented, and Profoundly Inequitable Model

The financing of the Congolese health sector currently rests on a highly unstable and dysfunctional three- pillar structure: an absent state, heavily overburdened households, and international donors with fluctuating, vertical priorities. The Congolese state allocates approximately 5% of its national budget to health—a figure critically below the 15% minimum mandate signed by African heads of state in the Abuja Accord. This envelope, already profoundly insufficient, is heavily absorbed by central administrative overhead in Kinshasa, leaving virtually nothing for rural health centers, district hospitals, or frontline dispensaries. Deprived of operational budgets, local facilities lack any financial autonomy, forcing clinicians to improvise daily with derisory means.

This massive state deficit is directly compensated for by the households themselves. It is estimated that out- of-pocket payments directly account for over 40% of total national health expenditures. For an average family, a short hospital admission represents immediate financial ruin. The cost of a prescription or emergency transport pushes entire families into chronic debt, forcing them to sacrifice other fundamental needs like food or education. Meanwhile, international aid, though substantial, remains volatile and uncoordinated. It is heavily directed toward vertical programs targeting specific infectious diseases (HIV, tuberculosis, malaria) according to external donor agendas, ignoring the horizontal reinforcement of baseline health systems. When these external grants expire, the fragile local structures built around them collapse entirely, due to a total lack of national integration or institutional handover.

Refunding Healthcare Finance on Principles of Solidarity and Justice

To exit this structural impasse, a radical financial reform is required. It must be built upon three non- negotiable pillars:

• **Health as a National Budgetary Priority:** Enact mandatory legislative commitments to progressively increase the state budget allocation toward health.

• **Institutional Risk-Pooling and Solidarity:** Move away from individual out-of-pocket models toward a national system where contributions are based on financial capacity, and care is delivered strictly based on clinical need.

• **The Total Eradication of Direct Point-of-Care Fees:** Transform direct cash payment at the point of service from the standard baseline norm into a rare exception.

This paradigm shift must begin by meeting the 15% Abuja Accord target within the national budget.

Achieving this threshold would safely cover healthcare worker salaries, maintain physical infrastructure, secure a continuous supply of essential generic medicines, and fund large-scale preventative health campaigns. Parallel to this, the progressive implementation of Universal Health Coverage (UHC) must serve as our primary structural engine. This framework will legally guarantee free primary healthcare—including consultations, maternal and neonatal care, mandatory vaccinations, and emergency triage. This will be sustainably funded through a combination of general state revenues, mandatory social health insurance contributions from the formal public and private sectors, and innovative risk-pooling mechanisms designed for the informal sector, such as community-based mutual health funds and micro-contributions integrated into mobile money transactions.

The centralized administration of this new financial architecture will be managed by a National Health Solidarity Fund (NHSF), decentralized via proactive provincial branches. This institution will pull all state allocations and international donor streams into a unified, transparent national framework, ensuring strict financial traceability and complete alignment with local public health priorities.

Concrete Financial Instruments to Deploy Solidarity

The success of this transition depends on our capacity to activate modern, credible financial instruments:

• **Earmarked National Health Tax:** Implement a dedicated health levy applied to formal salaries, paired with mandatory corporate health solidarity contributions levied on highly profitable extractive industries (mining, oil), telecommunications networks, and financial institutions.

• **Mobile-Integrated Informal Contributions:** Leverage the high penetration of mobile telephony to design streamlined micro-insurance enrollment options tailored for informal workers and agricultural communities.

• **National Health Equalization Fund:** Establish a transparent redistribution mechanism to channel revenues from wealthier, resource-rich provinces toward the most vulnerable, geographically isolated, and impoverished health zones.

• **Health Budget Information System (HBIS):** Deploy an open, digital financial tracking system backed by mandatory independent annual audits, allowing real-time monitoring of all financial flows down to the facility level and institutionalizing community-led oversight.

• **Health Compact DRC:** Enact a binding strategic framework with international donors to legally enforce the alignment of all external funding streams with the national health policy, ending vertical fragmentation.

It is no longer acceptable for a health system to impose its heaviest financial burden on those who possess the least, precisely at the moment when their physical and social vulnerability is at its peak. National solidarity ceases to be an abstract moral ideal and becomes a concrete institutional reality when every citizen contributes according to their financial means and receives high-quality care according to their clinical needs. Such an architecture requires unyielding political courage, transparent institutions, and a shared commitment to reposition health at the very center of our social contract. This financial revolution, to be sustainable, demands an entirely renewed, inclusive, and decentralized governance model—the major challenge we will analyze in the next part of this book.

PART II:

A VISION FOR A MODERN HEALTH SYSTEM

From Diagnostic Assessment to Transformative Ambition

The in-depth analysis of structural dysfunctions within the healthcare system of the Democratic Republic of the Congo, presented in the first part of this work, cannot remain a sterile academic critique. It must serve as the absolute foundation for an urgent call to action, a baseline launching pad toward a systemic refounding that has become completely unavoidable. Given the sheer scale of the institutional and operational deficits exposed, it would be dangerously illusory to rely on temporary stopgap fixes or superficial bureaucratic realignments.

What the DRC requires today is a radical change of direction, guided by an endogenous vision, deeply anchored in our local realities and propelled by our collective aspirations.

The Foundations of an Endogenous and Pragmatic Blueprint

The Democratic Republic of the Congo possesses an abundance of human capital and highly inspiring local community dynamics. Our population, overwhelmingly young, overflows with initiative, intelligence, and a unique capacity for resilience. The immense logistical and geographical challenges posed by our vast territory, rather than paralyzing us, must serve as a catalyst for localized, context-adapted innovation. Furthermore, our frontline healthcare professionals, though historically marginalized from central policy decisions, represent an incredible asset for systemic reconstruction, having had their clinical skills forged in adversity. It is from these unique internal strengths that a new national health strategy must emerge.

This manifests as a renewed social contract, binding the state, medical professionals, and the entire citizenry within a framework of shared constitutional responsibility. This pact cannot be reduced to a symbolic political declaration; it must constitute a legally binding, structural commitment founded on justice, regional coherence, and operational sustainability, capable of restoring public trust and meeting the real epidemiological needs of our populations.

Four Strategic Priorities for Deep Systemic Overhaul

The structural transformation of the Congolese health sector rests on four essential axes, designed as interconnected levers:

1. **Universal Territorial Access:** The absolute eradication of regional health inequities, guaranteeing every citizen an equal right to high-quality healthcare regardless of their geographic location, from urban centers to the most enclaved rural sectors.

2. **Homogeneous Care Quality:** Institutionalizing clinical excellence as a non-negotiable norm across all facilities, ensuring that medical safety and evidence-based protocols are never dictated by a patient's socio-economic status.

3. **Workforce Revaluation and Protection:** Rebuilding the human resources framework by securing dignified salaries, continuous medical education, and safe working environments, without which no system reform can succeed.

4. **Solidarity-Based Sustainable Financing:** Deploying a transparent, predictable risk-pooling financial architecture that guarantees absolute protection against catastrophic health expenditures through a logic of redistributive justice.

A Coherent Architecture for Lasting Systemic Change

The following chapters translate these four strategic priorities into concrete operational models:

• **Chapter 6** focuses on the comprehensive reorganization of the medical territory, outlining a dynamic, functional grid of health facilities paired with clear tier referral mechanisms to secure rural healthcare delivery.

• **Chapter 7** targets the modernization of clinical practice through the standardization of national evidence- based protocols, the integration of context-adapted technologies (offline electronic records, satellite telemedicine), and strict biomedical engineering standards.

• **Chapter 8** outlines the structural conditions required to optimize our human capital, detailing professional accreditation systems, decentralized career tracking, and retention models for remote areas.

• **Chapter 9** exposes the institutional architecture of Universal Health Coverage (ASURDC), detailing its mixed financing streams, solidarity mechanisms, and community-led governance.

This vision does not belong to an unachievable utopia. It relies entirely on verified local capacities, a shared desire for change, and a progressive, structured roadmap. It does not seek to blindly copy imported Western models, nor does it seek to maintain a chronic, degrading dependency on international humanitarian aid. The ultimate objective is to build a sovereign, self-sufficient Congolese health system aligned with our national priorities and funded by our own economy. Public health is not a secondary sector policy; it is the ultimate indicator of social justice, a symbol of human dignity, and the engine of national cohesion. To strengthen care, protect our clinicians, and ensure financial fairness is to rebuild the very foundations of our state. The blueprint is drawn. The operational levers are ready. What is required now is political will and a determined, unified mobilization. The time for waiting is over; the moment has arrived to execute.

Chapter 6:

Establishing Nationwide Territorial Equity and Access

Territorial Justice: The Absolute Foundation of a Democratic Health System

It is completely unacceptable for an individual's life expectancy to be determined by their place of birth. This fundamental ethical principle must serve as the absolute center of the structural revision of the Congolese health sector. In a nation marked by regional disparities as pronounced as the Democratic Republic of the

Congo—extending from the dense, hyper-populated markets of Matete to the deep equatorial forests of Mambasa, and from the vast river networks of Kwilu to the high plateaus of Kasaï—realizing territorial equity constitutes a colossal logistical challenge, yet it remains completely non-negotiable.

At the present hour, geographic inequalities in health delivery are glaring. While certain urban centers possess relative access to baseline medical services, rural populations are routinely left with rudimentary practices entirely devoid of qualified professional assistance. In remote sectors, mothers continue to face childbirth illuminated by candles, completely isolated from emergency obstetric equipment or technical supervision. These deep disparities are neither the result of historical coincidence nor a natural fatality. They are the direct consequence of consecutive, top-down political choices that have historically ignored the imperative of territorial justice.

A Fragmented Health System Operating at Multiple Speeds

The Congolese health infrastructure suffers from a highly dangerous state of fragmentation. Human, technological, and financial resources are overwhelmingly concentrated in a few urban centers, specifically within Kinshasa, while rural and border regions are structurally under-equipped, medically isolated, and frequently abandoned. Over the decades, health facilities have been constructed without any centralized planning, dictated by uncoordinated international NGO projects, localized political interests, or random private initiatives. This absolute lack of demographic orchestration has generated absurd redundancies in certain urban zones, leaving immense rural swaths in total medical desertification.

Staff allocations follow a logic entirely disconnected from the epidemiological realities of the ground. Dispatching a newly graduated physician or nurse into an enclaved health zone without providing functional staff housing, safe working conditions, or basic logistical support is an administrative failure that organizes their immediate departure. This chronic instability destroys the continuity of care and drives deep professional disengagement. Furthermore, the hyper-centralization of administrative decisions in Kinshasa paralyzes local adaptation. Public health strategies designed in central ministries rarely reflect the real operational constraints of distant provinces, widening the chasm between bureaucratic directives and the lived experience of rural communities.

Constructing a Health Network Rooted in Spatial Equity

To establish a truly equitable health system, we must radically break away from these historical failures. Guaranteeing every citizen—whether they reside in Lubefu, Bukama, or Shabunda—functional access to high- quality care requires an absolute structural reorganization built around three baseline principles:

• **The 5-Kilometer Proximity Mandate:** No village or community across the national territory should be located further than five kilometers from an operational primary health center. This proximity cannot be a hollow metric; it implies the permanent availability of essential generic drugs and continuous staffing.

• **Operational Secondary Referral Hubs:** Every rural health zone must possess an operational general referral hospital capable of managing emergency obstetric, surgical, and medical complications, eliminating dangerous long-distance transfers.

• **Differentiated Logistical Solutions:** Deploy customized, pragmatic mobility systems to overcome geographical barriers, including off-road 4x4 mobile clinics, medicalized river barges for enclaved riverine networks, and continuous satellite-linked tele-triage tools.

System governance must be deeply decentralized, responsible, and rigorously regulated. While the central ministry retains the statutory mandate to define national standards, regulate procurement, and ensure macro- financial equity, the actual planning and execution of health policies must be entirely devolved to the provinces and local health zones. Local health zones must become autonomous operational units with clear public health targets and budgets, evaluated strictly on verified clinical outcomes. Finally, absolute transparency and active community co-management must serve as the ultimate guardians of system credibility. All facility performance metrics must be made public, and Local Health Development Committees (CODESA) must be legally empowered with real budgets and oversight authority to drive a continuous cycle of local improvement.

Solid Operational Tools for Sustainable Territorial Realignment

Translating this territorial vision into a permanent reality relies on deploying modern operational instruments:

- **Real-Time Digital Health Mapping:** Deploy a comprehensive digital health map utilizing GPS and mobile technologies to track the exact location, staffing, and operational capacity of every facility, guiding all future capital infrastructure deployments.

- **Strict Pyramidal Referral Architecture:** Enforce a transparent, multi-tier health delivery pyramid where primary care centers manage baseline triage, general district hospitals handle secondary complications, and University Hospital Centers (CHU) focus exclusively on highly complex pathologies, fully fluidified by a national reference and counter-reference protocol.

- **National Mobile Health Service (NMHS):** Establish a specialized, state-funded mobile health service to rapidly deploy highly equipped, multi-disciplinary clinical teams into enclaved territories, post-conflict zones, or areas experiencing sudden epidemiological outbreaks.

- **Performance-Based Provincial Financing:** Restructure fiscal transfers to health zones, linking a significant portion of their operational budgets directly to verified health outcomes, such as vaccination coverage increases, maternal mortality reductions, and patient transit times.

- **Cross-Sectoral Development Integration:** Systematically align health zone strategies with parallel infrastructure developments: road rehabilitation, clean water access projects, rural electrification networks, and educational planning.

Overhauling the health sector goes far beyond a simple technocratic adjustments: it is a profound act of state building. Where a functional health center is missing, the state is invisible. Where human lives are lost due to a lack of basic primary care, the Republic is failing its constitutional promise. Restoring territorial equity across our healthcare delivery is the ultimate method to re-establish the presence of the state, restore civic trust, and strengthen national unity. This historic work cannot be evaluated from ministerial offices in Kinshasa; it will be measured in forgotten villages, deep rural clinics, and marginalized urban informal settlements. It is in the eyes of a reassured mother and the survival of a vulnerable child that the new Republic we aspire to build will manifest: a nation that is genuinely present for every citizen, everywhere.

Chapter 7:

Reinventing Medicine: Quality, Technology, and Protocol Standardization

A Technological Paradox Exposing an Institutional Emergency

"In my village, we have enough mobile network coverage to stream videos on TikTok, but we cannot contact a physician in an emergency." This observation, shared with a mixture of irony and despair by a frontline rural nurse, highlights a profound contradiction within our society: while modern telecommunications technology has penetrated deeply into the territory, it remains entirely unutilized to meet baseline human needs. This striking paradox underscores the urgent necessity for a thoughtful, systematic modernization of the

Congolese health system—conceived not as the blind importation of high-cost, fragile Western technology, but as a sober, realistic, and profoundly human adaptation of modern tools to our specific local realities.

In a nation characterized by extreme geographical constraints—unpaved roads that turn impassable during rainy seasons, vast river networks difficult to navigate, and complex, enclaved terrains—technological deployment must be directly adapted to the physical environment. A high-tech digital laboratory in Lubumbashi can never compensate for the absolute absence of basic medical records in Basankusu, where clinical consultations continue to be written on loose sheets of paper, guaranteeing the loss of patient history and zero continuity of care.

Severe Technical Deficits Conveying Heavy Human Costs

The chronic technological deficits within our health facilities are not mere administrative inconveniences; they directly translate into massive, avoidable human mortality. The absence of a standardized health information system completely paralyzes clinical traceability, delays the detection of epidemic outbreaks, and compromises the macro-planning of national health campaigns. Critical baseline vital statistics—such as births, maternal deaths, and real-time medical stock levels—are routinely inaccurate, incomplete, or completely absent from local registries.

Medical devices, when procured or donated, are frequently unsuited for local conditions or rapidly fall out of service. Our facilities are littered with broken ultrasound machines left non-functional due to voltage fluctuations, offline microscopes missing replacement bulbs for months, and a total absence of basic computers even within central district health offices. These technical failures directly compromise diagnostic safety and place an immense psychological burden on clinicians. In rural zones, community health workers represent the only link between the population and the formal medical network, yet they operate in absolute information isolation, lacking basic communication tools to report epidemiological alerts or request emergency clinical support. Consequently, life-threatening drug stockouts are only detected when they are already absolute, forcing medicine to remain entirely reactive, and leaving preventative healthcare completely marginalized.

Deploying Frugal, Human-Centered Medical Technology

Technology must never be pursued as an independent ideological goal; it must serve strictly as a tool to reinforce the safety and humanity of medical delivery. Modernizing rural healthcare does not mean equipping village clinics with complex surgical robotics, but rather providing frontline providers with simple, robust, and highly adapted clinical tools designed alongside the clinicians themselves.

The digitalization of care can be executed progressively without requiring heavy industrial infrastructure. A solar-powered tablet, a localized electronic medical record application that operates entirely offline, and a secure SMS-based data transmission system are entirely sufficient to immediately establish clinical traceability, patient tracking, and absolute continuity of care. To be effective, macro health planning must rely on verified, real-time data. Decentralized digital dashboards, early-warning epidemiological algorithms, and predictive supply chain software will allow governance to transition from a reactive crisis state to proactive, predictive management. From a clinical standpoint, national protocols must be translated into clear, highly visual, and easily comprehensible formats, translated into our national languages and accessible across lightweight digital channels (offline apps, SMS networks, visual charts). A thoughtful standardization of care does not paralyze a clinician's skills; on the contrary, it provides a safe clinical baseline that protects the patient while empowering professional judgment.

Furthermore, the communication loop between the health system and the community can be immediately transformed by basic digital tools: automated voice messages reminding mothers of infant vaccination schedules, rapid public health alerts broadcasted via localized community radio networks, and short toll-free codes to allow citizens to report drug stockouts. Every tool deployed must be structurally built to withstand the physical realities of our territory: high heat, pervasive dust, extreme electrical instability, and non-specialized handling. Technology must remain intuitive, highly reliable, and co-designed by the frontline workers who use it daily.

An Adaptable National Technological and Engineering Blueprint

Realizing this clinical and technological modernization requires building four solid institutional foundations:

- **Unified National EMR Architecture:** Establish a single National Digital Medical Record system linked to a simple patient identifier (encrypted QR code, personal ID number, or biometric print) that is fully readable locally offline, securely synchronized nationally, and activated strictly via patient consent.

- **Universal Free Tele-Triage Network:** Implement a state-supported, free satellite-linked telemedicine framework utilizing portable diagnostic kits to allow remote rural nurses to instantly upload clinical images and data to specialized physicians in provincial centers for real-time support.

- **Frugal and Standardized Device Procurement:** Enact a strict national standardization policy for medical devices, restricting procurement to robust, energy-efficient equipment with low maintenance requirements, paired with mandatory digital training modules delivered via accessible channels (WhatsApp networks, localized audio tutorials).

- **Provincial Biomedical Engineering Hubs:** Create fully funded biomedical engineering and maintenance centers within each province, ensuring that no diagnostic tool remains offline due to a lack of spare parts or technical expertise. Preventative maintenance must be treated as a core national security priority.

Modernizing Congolese medicine does not mean chasing innovation for the sake of novelty. It means placing technological intelligence directly at the service of human life, clinical safety, and operational efficiency, within a spirit of simplicity, sobriety, and profound respect for local realities. As a clinician in Kabeya Kamwanga emphasized: "We do not need advanced robotics; we need reliable clinical reference points." That is the true challenge. The machine must never replace the human touch;

it must support, protect, and amplify it. In this synergy between clinical know-how and robust technology, community health is strengthened, diagnostic rigor is democratized, and public trust is permanently restored. The modern medicine we are building will not be an imported luxury showcase; it will be tangible, accessible, sovereign, and profoundly Congolese.

Chapter 8:

Empowering Human Resources: Training, Status, and Recognition

The Human Capital: The Forgotten Foundation of Healthcare Delivery

When discussions turn to the modernization of a health system, the collective imagination tends to focus heavily on physical infrastructure, advanced diagnostic imaging technologies, or the integration of complex digital software. Yet, behind every single clinical intervention, every successful delivery, and every child vaccinated stands an individual human being. A lone nurse watching over a remote clinic in the mountains of South Kivu; a general practitioner delivering surgical care within a conflict-affected zone; a community health officer traveling kilometers on foot to educate and screen families in isolated villages: these women and men embody the beating heart of our healthcare delivery. Without their daily commitment, no medical apparatus, no matter how technologically advanced, can function.

Yet, the institutional, social, and economic recognition granted to our workforce remains profoundly inadequate given their critical role. The pervasive absence of formal employment contracts, highly erratic salary payments, a total lack of structured career advancement, and hierarchical relationships frequently marked by administrative indifference are not minor bureaucratic anomalies. They expose a deep, structural crisis of our national human capital that threatens the collapse of the entire system.

Structural Vulnerabilities in Human Resource Management

The primary vulnerability of our health system lies in the precarious legal and financial status of its clinicians. Thousands of healthcare workers practice for years without a formal civil service appointment, without basic occupational safety nets, and without any pension rights. As a health worker in Tshikapa describes: "I have been practicing on the frontline for eight years without a formal contract. When I fall ill, I must pay for my own medical treatment out of my empty pocket." This precariousness is a systemic operational failure.

Furthermore, there is a total absence of transparent professional development pathways. Promotion tracks are opaque, unmapped, or completely non-existent.

Specialized medical education remains heavily restricted to those who possess the independent financial means to relocate to Kinshasa or go abroad. Staff allocations follow arbitrary administrative logics, dispatching young clinicians into isolated rural zones without providing basic housing, functional clinical tools, or familial support structures. Baseline medical and nursing education remains overly theoretical and disconnected from the epidemiological and cultural realities of our communities. Rural clinical rotations, when they occur, are unguided and unsupported. Critical core competencies—including the patient-provider relationship, medical bioethics, digital health tools, and localized health crisis management—are routinely marginalized. Finally, a dangerous chasm separates frontline clinicians from academic research and central decision-makers. Data collected by frontline workers is uploaded into central systems without ever being synthesized or returned to the local teams to improve practice, and local clinical innovations are systematically ignored by central directorates, paralyzing the growth of a field-driven medical science.

A Comprehensive Revaluation of the Healthcare Workforce

The first step toward systemic reconstruction requires establishing a clear, legally protected, and highly motivating professional framework for all healthcare categories. This requires four structural components:

- **Formal Statutory Contracts:** A mandatory formal state contract for every active healthcare professional, guaranteeing full integration into the national civil service registry.

- **Transparent Remuneration Grid:** A unified salary scale based on verified qualifications, objective years of experience, and real clinical responsibility.

- **Mandatory Hardship Allowances:** Substantial, guaranteed financial allowances and housing packages specifically dedicated to those practicing in rural or high-risk territories.

- **Decentralized Rights to Continuing Education:** A statutory right to continuous professional education, fully decoupled from geographic location or personal connections.

Parallel to this, baseline medical and nursing curricula must undergo comprehensive reform, integrating robust, practical modules focused on community health, public health management, medical ethics, and digital tools, paired with highly structured and fully funded rural clinical rotations. Continuing professional education must be transformed into a core pillar of the career path—accessible, completely free of charge, and modular. A multilingual national digital platform must deliver high-quality clinical training content online and offline, ensuring equal professional advancement whether a clinician is practicing in Goma, Idiofa, Bukavu, or Boende.

True recognition, however, goes beyond financial compensation and digital courses. It requires celebrating and systematically scaling the operational innovations developed by clinicians on the ground. This implies replacing punitive bureaucratic evaluations with constructive, formative annual peer reviews, organizing provincial clinical exchange circles, building localized medical libraries, and institutionalizing national health workforce celebration days. Finally, we must actively fund and rehabilitate field-driven medical research.

Supporting scientific publications by district clinicians, providing state grants for local health center innovations, and recognizing empirical field knowledge as a vital source of medical science are the fundamental prerequisites to building a sustainable, proud, and self-sufficient health workforce.

Solid Institutional Frameworks for Lasting Career Transformation

To anchor this human capital strategy within a permanent legal architecture, specific structural bodies must be created:

- **Specialized Medical and Nursing Colleges:** Establish autonomous professional colleges for each cadre (physicians, nurses, midwives, biomedical technicians) tasked with managing clinical accreditation, continuously auditing workforce competencies, and tailoring career paths to provincial realities.

- **National CPD Credit Tracking System:** Enact a mandatory National Continuing Professional Development (CPD) credit framework, requiring every practicing clinician to acquire 20 to 30 certified credits annually through hybrid courses, directly unlocking promotions, geographical mobility, and senior clinical roles.

- **National Council for Health Workforce Development:** Found a centralized governance council uniting the Ministries of Health, Higher Education, and Finance alongside professional orders, health unions, and NGOs to ensure long-term alignment between medical training output and the real epidemiological needs of our territories.

It is entirely possible to construct physical hospital buildings, procure fleets of modern ambulances, and deploy advanced health management software. However, without highly competent, motivated, protected, and respected human beings to animate them, any system reform will collapse. Our healthcare workers are the true builders of our national sanitary sovereignty. This sovereignty cannot be decreed by administrative signatures; it is constructed daily through safe clinical acts, delivered within dignified working conditions, and sustained by mutual trust between the clinician and the state. Valuing our workforce is not an act of political charity; it is a profound matter of justice and the absolute prerequisite for system refounding. Providing a nurse with the tools to practice safely, a community health worker with the means to prevent disease, and a physician with the opportunity to grow professionally without having to flee their country is how we restore the human heart of Congolese healthcare.

Chapter 9:

Universal Health Coverage and Financial Solidarity

Escaping the Deep Injustice of Direct Out-of-Pocket Payments

For the vast majority of citizens in the Democratic Republic of the Congo, health is perceived as a commercial luxury conditioned entirely by immediate financial capacity, rather than an inalienable right guaranteed by the national community. Daily, ordinary scenes across our territory illustrate this silent human tragedy: a mother forced to sell her remaining livestock in Kenge to pay for an emergency cesarean section; a feverish child left completely without medical attention for days in Beni because their parents have an empty wallet; a clinically recovered patient physically detained inside a hospital ward in Kisangani for consecutive weeks due to an unpaid medical invoice.

These situations are not isolated anomalies; they highlight the absolute collapse of a baseline social principle: equal access to healthcare independent of economic status. In a broken system where every clinical act is treated as a commercial transaction, poverty transforms into a physical death sentence, and extreme inequity settles in as the baseline norm. It is not merely pathogens and diseases that destroy human lives across our nation, but the total absence of institutionalized financial solidarity, the deep historical withdrawal of the state from social protections, and the absolute void left around vulnerable families who possess zero health insurance, zero social safety nets, and zero institutional recourse.

When Access to Healthcare Operates as a Blind Social Lottery

The financing architecture of the Congolese health sector, as it stands today, operates on profoundly unjust mechanisms. Clinical quality and healthcare access are never determined by real medical need or the principle of universal human value, but by a chaotic series of random external factors: one's city of birth, social status, personal political connections, or the pure luck of encountering a benevolent clinician. This institutional layout turns healthcare into a blind lottery.

Within this framework, direct out-of-pocket cash payment at the point of service stands as an insuperable structural barrier. Medical consultations, diagnostic tests, and vital prescriptions are treated as highly priced commodities subject to immediate financial clearance. Consequently, life-saving clinical decisions are systematically delayed, scaled down, or entirely canceled by families. This forces our population to resort to dangerous self-medication, unregulated informal parallel markets, or spiritual escapes, fleeing from a formal health apparatus that should be their primary shield of protection. This failure goes beyond epidemiological metrics: it rapidly erodes civic trust in national institutions, fractures the social fabric, and feeds a continuous cycle of multi-generational poverty, exclusion, and deep public mistrust. We must radically break away from this commercial model through an absolute structural refounding based on a single baseline truth: health is a public good, not a market commodity.

Rebuilding Healthcare around the Core Engine of Solidarity

Faced with the profound injustice of the current system, a powerful structural alternative must be deployed: a national framework for Universal Health Coverage. This model rests on a simple, non-negotiable axiom: access to healthcare must be entirely decoupled from individual income and linked strictly to national citizenship. In a Republic fully engaged in its reconstruction, health must be guaranteed to every citizen as the absolute rock of social justice.

The delivery of free essential healthcare must never be viewed as an act of periodic political charity or temporary humanitarian generosity. It must be institutionalized as the visible, legally binding manifestation of a national pact of solidarity. It represents a formal recognition of the absolute, equal value of every human life across our territory, completely independent of one's socio-economic status, income tier, or geographic province.

The Architecture of the Universal Health Insurance System (ASURDC)

Establishing a comprehensive, resilient system of Universal Health Coverage in the DRC, which we designate as ASURDC, requires building a highly coherent, transparent, and financially sustainable institutional architecture structured around three non-negotiable pillars:

1. **An Autonomous National Solidarity Fund System:** Create a highly credible, independent National Health Solidarity Fund managed via a shared governance structure uniting the state, healthcare professional orders, and civil society

representatives. This institution will be legally mandated to publish detailed, publicly accessible annual financial reports to secure complete institutional accountability.

2. **A Guaranteed Essential Package of Care:** Define a comprehensive, legally protected baseline care package guaranteed free of charge to every citizen, encompassing all emergency triage, maternal and neonatal care, complete childhood vaccinations, management of common endemic pathologies, and full access to essential generic medicines. This package will be continuously updated based on evolving national epidemiological trends.

3. **A Diversified and Progressive Risk-Pooling Model:** Deploy a robust, mixed financing stream that combines mandatory social health insurance contributions from formal public and private sector salaries; an earmarked national health solidarity tax levied on highly profitable corporate sectors (extractive mining and oil industries, telecommunications, banking networks) and luxury goods; direct targeted state subsidies to fully cover vulnerable demographics; and streamlined micro-contribution frameworks designed for the informal and agricultural sectors using localized community mutual funds and integrated mobile money transaction levies.

This architecture embodies a central principle of social justice: each contributes according to their financial capacity, and each receives care strictly according to their clinical need. It redefines health as a collective national asset protected by a unified network of mutual aid, rebuilding civic trust in public institutions.

A Progressive, Transparent, and Participatory Deployment Plan

The national deployment of ASURDC cannot be achieved overnight through a single administrative decree. It requires a graduated, highly calculated rollout plan, anchored in rigorous pilot phases across selected test provinces to continuously evaluate risk-pooling mechanics, audit local supply chains, collect provider feedback, and fine-tune operational software prior to national scaling.

System governance must be deeply participatory and transparent. Local Health Management Boards must be created within each health zone, composed of real users, local clinicians, and civil society representatives, legally empowered to track budgets, audit facility performance, and manage formal patient grievance systems. These local boards will act as the frontline guardians of civic oversight, ensuring that public resources directly serve patient health rather than bureaucratic overhead. Furthermore, a permanent culture of independent scientific evaluation must be institutionalized through continuous tracking of key health outcome metrics, mandatory external clinical audits, and public impact studies, ensuring the system remains responsive, transparent, and fully accountable to the nation.

A Project of National Society, Not a Mere Bureaucratic Adjustment

We must state this truth with absolute clarity: universal health protection is not a secondary luxury reserved exclusively for wealthy Western nations. It is a baseline political choice, the ultimate indicator of a state's democratic maturity, and the primary engine of long-term human and economic development. It is a profound reconfiguration of the social contract between the state and the citizen.

Every mother who delivers her child safely and free of charge in Kalemie, every child cured of malaria without plunging their parents into debt in Mbandaka, and every informal worker protected against catastrophic health costs in Bunia represents a concrete victory for our society. This project is the ultimate vector for true national reconciliation. It makes the protection of the state tangible, proving to our population that the Republic cares for their lives, protects their families, and leaves no citizen behind.

Investing in universal health solidarity must never be misconstrued as a dead economic cost or an unsustainable budgetary burden. On the contrary, it represents the most strategic, ethical, and economically productive investment a nation can undertake. A healthy population is a population that learns effectively, works productively, innovates continuously, and sustains long-term civil peace. It liberates families from the terror of sudden financial ruin, restores human dignity to the center of national life, and transforms solidarity into our primary national engine. We must seize this historic turning point. This moment cannot be delayed or reduced to symbolic promises. It demands bold legislative ambition, absolute financial rigor, and unwavering political commitment. Constructing an equitable health system funded via collective solidarity is the true cornerstone of our future: a unified, strong, and deeply humane Republic.

PART III:

STRUCTURAL IMPLEMENTATION BLUEPRINT

Translating Strategic Vision into Verifiable Public Health Outcomes

The ultimate test of any public health strategy does not lie in the elegant design of its theoretical vision, but in the institutional capacity to translate political intentions into verifiable, long-term health outcomes on the ground. Despite a multitude of national health strategies, master plans, and health updates drafted over the history of the Democratic Republic of the Congo, our nation has frequently experienced severe implementation failures. These failures have been driven primarily by the historic absence of robust execution mechanisms, a total lack of transparent independent evaluations, and weak, unstable institutional frameworks susceptible to political fluctuations.

The Four Absolute Non-Negotiable Conditions for Lasting Reform

To ensure that this strategic blueprint does not remain a dead letter, its national execution must strictly adhere to four institutional requirements:

1. **Resilient and De-Politicized Institutions:** The creation of legally protected, permanent public health bodies and statutory funds capable of steering long-term reforms entirely independent of political transitions, electoral cycles, or ministerial changes.

2. **Rigorous, Multi-Level Decentralized Governance:** A crystal-clear operational alignment between the central, provincial, and local health zone authorities, establishing absolute budgetary autonomy at the base while avoiding both paralyzing hyper-centralization and uncoordinated, chaotic regional implementation.

3. **Continuous Data-Driven Progress Audits:** Institutionalizing real-time digital monitoring loops utilizing shared, transparent performance metrics to allow health administrators to immediately detect operational deficits and adjust resource allocation.

4. **Institutionalized Civic Co-Architecture:** Elevating the citizen and local civil

society from passive health consumers into active, legally empowered co-architects of health delivery, embedding bottom-up accountability into the core of the system.

Activating the Four Primary Operational Levers for Execution

Transitioning from strategic planning to concrete field execution requires the immediate activation of four structural levers:

• **Authentic Decentralization of Human and Fiscal Resources:** Legally transfer real financial envelopes and human resource management autonomy directly to the provincial health directorates, ensuring local zones can react dynamically to their specific epidemiological crises.

• **Deploying Modern, Centralized Digital Dashboard Management:** Fully equip all health tiers with integrated health information software to ensure public health choices are driven strictly by verified scientific evidence rather than political guesswork.

• **Statutory Civic Oversight and Social Audits:** Legalize the oversight authority of community health boards, giving citizens the statutory right to perform open public audits of local health budgets and facility supply chains.

• **Securing a Highly Stable, Transparent Legislative Framework:** Enact comprehensive public health legislation to provide total fiscal transparency, protect healthcare funding streams from embezzlement, and secure an open, permanent dialogue with all medical orders, unions, and financial partners.

The era of hollow political promises and endless paper reports is permanently behind us. The ultimate success of this healthcare reform will never be measured by the beauty of its strategic documents, but through the real, daily clinical conditions experienced by our patients and frontline clinicians. This structural transformation depends entirely on the capacity of the state to execute an organized, coherent, and deeply transparent public action centered on the real life of its population. This is the precise methodology through which this healthcare blueprint will transform into sustainable, equitable, and profoundly human progress for the entire nation.

Chapter 10:

Governance, Applied Research, and Change Leadership

Building an Accountable and Transformative Governance Framework

The comprehensive overhaul of a national health system cannot be sustained by catchy political slogans, superficial rebranding, or isolated, short-term pilot projects without an institutional tomorrow. It requires building an ironclad, highly structured governance architecture—conceived not as a passive administrative checklist, but as a powerful engine of collective mobilization, a strategic organizing force capable of maintaining long-term direction, uniting disparate clinical actors, and guaranteeing absolute operational continuity over decades.

Managing public health is not about imposing an abstract, top-down technocratic agenda from ministerial offices in Kinshasa. It requires the active coordination of a highly complex, fragmented ecosystem of providers, donors, and regional authorities, orchestrating their diverse interactions within a single, coherent national framework. This governance must be entirely anchored in field reality, fueled by transparent scientific facts, and heavily protected against arbitrary administrative choices. In an environment oversaturated with fluctuating personal opinions and political pressures, system choices must rest firmly on verified data, objective clinical outcomes, and transparent performance metrics.

Strategic Change Leadership as the Engine of Operational Efficiency

The operational efficiency of change leadership relies on three non-negotiable pillars: the absolute availability of verified health data, total clarity of key performance indicators, and complete institutional transparency in the auditing of public health outcomes. Steering a system without real-time, accurate epidemiological data is equivalent to navigating an ocean completely blind. Setting health targets without deploying verifiable measurement tools is an admission of zero institutional responsibility. Finally, ignoring the immediate necessity for structural course corrections when severe operational deficits are exposed condemns the entire national framework to permanent stagnation.

Effective public health leadership can never be executed as a solitary bureaucratic exercise. It must actively leverage a dense, decentralized network of diverse stakeholders: from frontline rural nurses to provincial health directors, and from academic researchers to international technical partners and the citizens themselves. True, sustainable ownership of system change and the absolute democratic legitimacy of administrative decisions emerge exclusively from this diversity of institutional engagement.

Deep Structural Faults within the Current Governance Apparatus

At the present hour, the governance of our health sector faces profound, systemic paralysis. Central ministries, international technical agencies, and humanitarian NGOs operate within isolated, hyper-fragmented silos entirely devoid of centralized coordination. Massive financial and human resources are routinely wasted on redundant, overlapping regional projects, while baseline national health priorities are constantly realigned to match the arbitrary fiscal cycles of foreign donors rather than the real epidemiological and medical needs of the Congolese population.

Furthermore, the central health authority suffers from a severe deficit in strategic leadership. The historic absence of a permanent, unified state organ capable of enforcing long-term policy coherence prevents the emergence of a sustainable reform dynamic. As for the decentralization framework, it remains a hollow fiction restricted to legislative papers, completely paralyzed by a total lack of localized operational budgets and a clear absence of political will from the center. Concurrently, medical and public health research remains entirely disconnected from the operational realities of frontline clinics. Research operates as the exclusive, high-cost privilege of a few urban academic institutions in Kinshasa, lacking any functional feedback loops with rural clinical practices or systematic integration into the design of national health laws. Valuable localized health data is regularly generated on the ground, but it is never shared effectively across provinces or utilized to guide central executive choices.

Reconstructing Strategic Governance to Meet Continental Challenges

To overcome these severe systemic blockages, a profound structural reconstruction must be executed. The national Ministry of Public Health must fully reclaim its legal mandate as the sovereign strategic orchestrator of the entire sector. To realize this, we must urgently legislate the creation of a permanent Secretariat for Cross- Sectoral Health Coordination, providing a dedicated institutional space to permanently align health strategy with parallel national policies: education, public finance, infrastructure, and local development. This will embed health across a transversal national architecture, breaking down historical bureaucratic silos.

The national health budget can no longer remain indexed to unpredictable, short-term foreign grants or sudden humanitarian crises. It must reflect a sovereign, long-term fiscal vision explicitly bound to the statutory mandates of Universal Health Coverage and protected by solid legislative funding streams. Concurrently, provincial directorates must be legally empowered with real, predictable financial envelopes, complete autonomy over local health zone planning, and the explicit statutory capacity to adapt national public health directives to their unique regional geographic and epidemiological specificities. Finally, we must institutionalize the mandatory organization of an annual National Health Governance Conference, tasked with delivering an unedited, fully transparent public audit detailing national health progress, financial flows, and operational failures.

A Robust Scientific and Data Infrastructure as a Catalyst for Change

A modernized, highly secure health information system is the absolute cornerstone of contemporary health governance. Fully digitalizing this information grid down to the most remote primary care dispensaries must be treated as a primary state security priority. This is not a basic data-entry exercise; it requires the secure cross-referencing and algorithmic analysis of real-time epidemiological metrics, fluidly integrated with civil registries, educational data, and national social security networks to build a comprehensive, multi-dimensional understanding of our population's health dynamics.

Concurrently, public health research must break out of its isolated academic towers. We must launch a specialized National Applied Research Fund dedicated exclusively to funding field-driven, operational health system questions, accelerating the discovery of localized solutions that can be immediately integrated into daily clinical practice. Promoting tight, mandatory collaborative networks between data scientists, clinical trialists, frontline providers, and executive policymakers is the only mechanism to transform science into a real engine of systemic change, rather than a factory for useless, unread bureaucratic reports.

Repositioning the Citizen at the Absolute Center of Health Governance

It is a dangerous illusion to attempt a profound system reform while excluding the active participation of the citizenry. The population must possess clear, legally protected channels to perform independent evaluations of public policies, report local medical corruptions or drug stockouts, and actively shape local health responses. This requires legally institutionalizing Community Health Governance Boards within every single health zone, launching secure, free digital health-vigilance platforms accessible to all, and enforcing simplified, legally binding administrative protocols to handle and resolve patient complaints rapidly.

This civic dimension of governance is not an optional democratic luxury. It is the ultimate mechanism to guarantee that defined public health priorities match the real needs of our communities, ensure that institutions are evaluated on concrete outcomes rather than bureaucratic paperwork, and allow operational errors to be corrected before they cost human lives. True health democracy thrives on absolute transparency, institutional responsibility, and radical inclusion. No public health reform can generate lasting effects without strong, unyielding, and highly agile change leadership. The noblest medical intentions, the largest financial investments, and the strongest international partnerships will remain entirely void of real-world impact if the system is steered without long-term coherence, moral courage, and clinical perseverance. Success depends entirely on building resilient public institutions capable of withstanding political transitions, establishing an institutional culture of performance judged on verified health outcomes, and sustaining a continuous political will decoupled from short-term electoral timelines. To govern public health today is to learn continuously from the field, listen to the base, adjust protocols without delay, and report outcomes with absolute honesty. A well-governed health system is the ultimate expression of a renewed social contract—founded on an unyielding respect for human life, absolute equality of constitutional rights, and total trust between the state and its citizens. It embodies the capacity of a nation to rise to its most fundamental sovereign responsibility.

GENERAL CONCLUSION:

REDESIGNING HEALTH, REBUILDING THE NATION

The Democratic Republic of the Congo can no longer be defined strictly by its deficits. Our nation embodies something far greater than a developing country navigating complex logistical challenges: it is a sovereign nation possessing an immense, unprecedented human and natural capital, reinforced by rich cultural diversity, an energetic youth demographic, and above all, the deep, resilient dignity of its citizens. Daily, working in the shadows of our territory, thousands of Congolese women and men invest their absolute energy into acts of medical care, education, community organizing, and social protection—frequently completely devoid of state resources, yet driven by an unyielding determination. It is to this quiet internal strength, this silent resilience, that our health system must respond: by delivering a medical framework that is safe, dignified, highly reliable, and profoundly human.

This book does not seek to present just another abstract technocratic proposal. It targets a far more ambitious horizon: it stands as a direct call for national commitment, a strategic map for executive alignment, and an operational tool to fuel a collective national vision where health is permanently redefined not as a secondary administrative service, but as the absolute pillar of our national commonwealth.

A Multifaceted Crisis Demanding a Comprehensive Transformation

The prolonged crisis of the Congolese health sector does not stem merely from a lack of physical tools or clinical envelopes. It is the direct reflection of a wider institutional fragility, marked by historically weak governance, severe structural territorial imbalances, and a dangerous chasm between the state and the population. Faced with this reality, short-term vertical programs or emergency humanitarian responses are completely obsolete. What our nation urgently requires is a deep, structural refounding—inscribed in long-term legislation, propelled by a coherent political will, and anchored in our shared national intelligence.

The Six Pillars of a Reconstructed National Health System

Throughout the chapters of this blueprint, six strategic axes have emerged, forming the dynamic engine of our national transformation:

1. **Proactive Strategic Planning:** Moving completely away from reactive crisis management toward predictive, data-driven planning that anticipates epidemiological shifts and directly aligns public health spending with verified field needs.

2. **Dignified Physical Environments:** Transforming our facilities into structurally safe, clean, solar- powered, and well-equipped environments, restoring public trust and respecting patient dignity.

3. **Standardized Clinical Excellence:** Eradicating multi-tier medicine by enforcing strict, evidence-based national clinical guidelines across all territories, ensuring diagnostic safety is independent of wealth.

4. **Workforce Empowerment and Protection:** Securing formal civil service contracts, dignified wages, comprehensive health insurance, and decentralized continuous medical education for our frontline clinicians.

5. **Redistributive Financial Solidarity:** Establishing Universal Health Coverage (ASURDC) funded via progressive cross-subsidization, tax levies on high-profit industries, and mobile risk-pooling, ensuring health is a fundamental right rather than a commercial commodity.

6. **Transparent Democratic Governance:** Repositioning the Ministry of Health as a sovereign strategic orchestrator, backed by dynamic digital dashboards and legally empowered community oversight boards to ensure total institutional accountability.

Health as a Unified Collective Responsibility

Overhauling our health architecture cannot be perceived as an isolated task exclusively assigned to the central state. It is a collective national responsibility that engages every sector of our society. The public authorities possess the binding constitutional duty to enforce a clear strategic vision and allocate the necessary national wealth. Frontline healthcare professionals must be recognized as the primary guardians of this transformation, supported in their refusal to yield to professional resignation. Our scientists and university researchers hold the responsibility to guide public policy choices through robust, independent operational data. Civil society organizations must remain intensely vigilant, operating as continuous forces of strategic proposal and public alert. Finally, the citizens themselves must actively reclaim their democratic power to demand institutional accountability and co-manage their local health zones. True reform is never dictated from the top; it is constructed from the base, rooted in the ownership of the users, the legitimacy of clinical practices, and the absolute transparency of public commitments.

Sanitary Sovereignty as Our Definitive Political Horizon

The structural transformation outlined within this work belongs neither to an unachievable dream nor to an unrealistic ambition. It is entirely reasonable and immediately executable, provided we operate under a single baseline economic truth: health is a high-return national investment, not a dead budgetary cost. A highly structured, equitable public health system generates powerful multi-sectoral dividends—stabilizing regional human capital, accelerating economic productivity, and heavily strengthening national security and social peace. We must permanently change our fiscal perspective. Health can no longer be treated as a secondary budget line item to be continuously restricted, but as a sovereign promise to be honored. Our goal is not to patch up a failing, broken apparatus, but to build, with intense lucidity and high ambition, a medical system worthy of the great nation we are destined to become.

We cannot afford to wait for perfect external conditions or complex global international treaties before we act. We must execute immediately, starting exactly where we are, maximizing the assets we currently possess, and moving forward with unyielding determination. Healthcare sovereignty is an inseparable component of national sovereignty. It is the ultimate reflection of the collective project carried by a Republic. A nation that safely protects the lives of its citizens affirms its humanity, its moral authority, and its sovereign capacity to self-govern while offering every human being a dignified existence.

Not a Final Conclusion, But a National Beginning

This text does not seek to close a public health discussion; it is designed to launch a vast national debate. It stands as an institutional lever, an operational reference point, and a tool for national convergence. Its true value will never reside in the elegance of the ideas it defends, but in the concrete legislative actions it inspires and the structural commitments it triggers across the territory. To our political decision-makers, it addresses a firm invitation to permanently break away from half-measures. To our frontline healthcare workers, it offers a discreet tribute to their central role and a call for absolute professional perseverance. To the Congolese population, it delivers a solemn promise: that an entirely different, safe, and dignified health system is fully within our reach, if we collectively choose to build it. Every single day counts. Every localized action, no matter how modest it may appear, represents a decisive victory against fatalism. What we sow today across our territory will determine not only the health of tomorrow, but the very nature of the society we choose to construct: a nation that is deeply just, profoundly humane, and structurally united, where health is no longer a commercial privilege, but a living, breathing reality for all.

BIBLIOGRAPHICAL REFERENCES

Foundational Official Publications and Reports

1. Ministry of Public Health, Hygiene and Prevention of the DRC (2022). *National Health Development Plan 2022–2026.* Kinshasa: Ministry of Health.

2. National Institute of Statistics (2023). *Statistical Yearbook 2023 – Socio-Sanitary Indicators.* Kinshasa: INS.

3. World Bank (2021).*Democratic Republic of the Congo Health Financing System Assessment: Challenges and Opportunities.* Technical Report No. 145632ZR. Washington D.C.: World Bank.

4. World Health Organization, Regional Office for Africa (2022). *Health Product Profile of the Democratic Republic of the Congo.* Brazzaville: WHO Afro.

Health Systems and Universal Coverage Frameworks

1. World Health Organization (2007). *Everybody's Business – Strengthening Health Systems to Improve Health Outcomes: WHO Framework for Action.* Geneva: WHO.

2. Commission on Social Determinants of Health (2008). *Closing the Gap in a Generation: Health Equity through Action on the Social Determinants of Health.* Geneva: WHO.

3. International Health Partnership (2013). *Joint Assessment of National Health Strategies and Plans: Technical Guidance for National and International Partners.* Geneva: WHO.

4. The Lancet Commission (2021). *The Path to Equitable and Resilient Health Systems in Sub-Saharan Africa.* The Lancet, 398(10308), 1395–1450.

Governance and Healthcare System Reform

1. Savedoff, W.D. & Smith, A.L. (2006). *Measuring Governance in the Health*

Sector. Center for Global Development, Working Paper No. 94. Washington D.C.: CGD.

2. Lewis, M. (2006). *Governance and Corruption in Public Health Care Systems.* Center for Global Development, Working Paper No. 78. Washington D.C.: CGD.

3. UNICEF, UNDP & WHO (2017). *Building Resilient Health Systems in Fragile Settings – A Framework for Action.* Geneva: WHO.

4. Transparency International (2006). *Global Corruption Report 2006: Special Focus on Corruption and the Health Sector.* London: Pluto Press.

Medical Research, Innovation, and Information Systems

1. Alliance for Health Policy and Systems Research (2012). *Health Systems Research: A Framework for Action.* Geneva: WHO.

2. Health Observatory for Central Africa (2021). *Annual Report 2021: Territorial Inequities in Healthcare Access across Central Africa.* Kinshasa: OSAC.

3. UNESCO (2022). *Science, Technology and Innovation in Africa: Global Report on Digital Health Innovations.* Paris: UNESCO.

Complementary Field Data and Qualitative Sources

1. Projet Congo Santé (2020–2023). *Internal Technical Archives: Strategy Notes, Draft Policies, and Multi- Stakeholder Consultation Minutes.* Kinshasa: Internal Project Repositories.

2. National Qualitative Field Assessments (2022–2023). *Comprehensive Compendium of Lived Experiences and In-Depth Interviews with Congolese Health System Actors*, comprising:

   ◦ 45 structured interviews with frontline healthcare professionals (physicians, nurses, midwives, community health workers).

   ◦ 32 interviews with local, provincial, and regional public health administrators.

◦ 28 bilateral interviews with international technical and financial partners.

◦ 60 detailed community focus groups with health facility users and community leaders.

3. Ministry of Plan and International Cooperation (2021). *National Growth and Poverty Reduction Strategy 2021–2025.* Kinshasa: MPCI.

4. Civil Society Health Forum DRC (2022). *Strategic Positioning of Civil Society on the Structural Reform of the Congolese Health System – Synthesis Report.* Kinshasa: FSCS.

5. National Episcopal Conference of the Congo (2021). *The Structural Contribution of Confessional and Faith-Based Health Networks to the Congolese Medical Grid: Assessment and Horizons.* Kinshasa: CENCO.

www.ingramcontent.com/pod-product-compliance
Lightning Source LLC
LaVergne TN
LVHW051130210926
848482LV00001B/45